Plant Based

Cookbook

Snack & Dessert

Plant Based Recipes for Healthy Mind and Body. A Kick-Start Guide to Eat and Live Your Best

By

Margaret McKinley

Table of Contents

Introduction

The veggie lover diet is generally known for is medical advantages, and specifically - weight reduction. Numerous people have experienced the veggie lover diet for the sole reason to get in shape, and have prevailing with regards to doing as such. On the off chance that you are looking for a sound and safe eating routine to get more fit, and are thinking about the vegetarian diet, you have to ask yourself: Is it safe? Is it astute? Is it feasible?

Is It Safe?

In the event that you experience the vegetarian diet in a reasonable, well-arranged way, you can be certain that it is both protected and solid. You have to guarantee that you are eating a wide range of nourishments consistently to guarantee that you are accepting ideal sustenance - however hello, you have to do this on any eating regimen. If you somehow managed to fall back on eating veggie lover low quality nourishment all the time, your wellbeing would clearly endure.

Veggie lover low quality nourishment incorporates parcel crisps, hot chips, without dairy chocolate and pieces of candy, alleged 'wellbeing bars' that are pressed with sugar, and so on. If you somehow managed to expend nourishments, for example, this all the time and eat them instead of your appropriate suppers, you are harming your body. Rather, you can select to make your own vegetarian preparing plans, for example, without dairy, low-sugar treats, brownies, cakes, oat and nut cuts, and so on., including dates, dried organic products, crisp natural products, nuts, coconut oil, extra-virgin olive oil and seeds. Experience your eating routine in a judicious and steady way, and give your body the supplements that it needs.

Is It Astute?

In the event that you have to shed pounds, the veggie lover diet is really one of the solid eating regimens that you can embrace to do as such. It is rash to decide on a craze diet that is low in Fat, low in supplements and leaves you feeling denied.

You can appreciate avocadoes, olive oil, nuts and seeds on this eating regimen - not at all like many accidents abstains from food today. You can likewise appreciate a scope of gourmet, solid cooking so you won't have to feel denied. By making your own heavenly and solid veggie lover heating plans, you are guaranteeing that you will stay glad and substance on this eating routine, as opposed to discouraged and grumpy.

So, if the veggie lover diet offers you a lot of sound supplements, gives your body adequate solid Fat s and doesn't leave you feeling denied, okay say that it is shrewd or indiscreet to wander down this pathway? I would state that it is savvy.

Is It Practical?

There are some long-haul veggie lovers who have been either on the vegetarian diet as long as they can remember or for a long time. These individuals are constantly thin and lean and have a sound, gleaming composition and a get-up-and-go that many are desirous of. Not at all like accident eats less, this eating regimen is reasonable. Why? You won't feel denied as there are numerous yummy alternatives to eat. You can appreciate a wide scope of lovely veggie lover heating plans or dinner plans, which are anything but difficult to discover in books, on the web, or from vegetarian formula digital books. The medical advantages of this eating regimen will cause you to understand that it is well-worth neglecting meat and dairy items. Many have done as such and are proceeding to do so today. Could this be you?

Weight reduction on the vegetarian diet is sheltered, savvy and economical. So maybe it is currently an opportunity to discard the entirety of your accident diet musings and ideas, and choose rather a sound, veggie lover way of life that will leave your life elements glad, solid and well-supported.

The discussion of whether the vegetarian diet is sound or unfortunate isn't new. Most of people will state that an individual who embraces veganism will be insufficient in basic supplements found distinctly in creature items, to be specific, creature-based Protein.

These people treasure the conviction that dairy milk will help keep their bones solid and that red meat will give basic Protein to their muscles.

Then again, there is a little minority of people (2% veggie lover and 5% vegan) who offer credit to the plant-based eating routine relieving their genuine medical issues, empowering them to lose overabundance weight, clearing up their skin and sensitivities, and giving them an astounding pizza.

So dependent on these two contrasts in assessments, how might one decide if the veggie lover diet is solid or undesirable? Everything comes down to, not matters of 'conclusion,' yet rather, on strong actualities, proof, contextual analyses and honest accounts of genuine individuals.

Meat Eaters Vs. Veggie Eaters

Various investigations demonstrate that eaters of red meat are bound to kick the bucket rashly than the individuals who eat almost no red meat. One US-based investigation of 120,000 individuals verified that eaters of red meat are 20% bound to pass on more youthful. The individuals who ate prepared meats routinely supported this sudden passing rate to a further 20% higher.

Then again, Michael F. Roizen, MD, infers that the individuals who change from eating meat items to veggie lover nourishments could without much of a stretch add at any rate 13 years to their life. Why? Veggie lovers eat less creature Fat and cholesterol, while vegetarians devour no creature Fat or cholesterol. Educator T. Colin. Campbell (raised on a dairy ranch) closes from his test look into program that a meat and without dairy diet can both avert and turn around 70-80% of infection!

Weight Reduction Evidence

Actuality: most meat and dairy items are high in Fat and calorie content. For instance, 100g of sheep contains around 294 calories and 21g of Fat (9% soaked) while 100g of cooked lentils contains just 128 calories and 6.5g of Fat (0.8g immersed). Sheep has 0g dietary fiber, while 100g of lentils contains 7.5g dietary fiber. Fiber causes you to feel more full for more.

Proof:

Angela Stokes (AKA 'Veggie lover Raw Food Goddess') lost over 154lbs (70kg) on the vegetarian crude nourishment diet. This astounding lady, once extremely chubby, validates her weight reduction and newly discovered vitality to the veggie lover crude nourishment diet and will not come back to the standard American DIRECTIONS for eating! Why? The medical advantages of the veggie lover diet (especially weight reduction for Angela's situation) are too incredible to even consider giving up. Angela received crude veganism medium-term and has never thought back since.

PHYSICAL BENEFITS

Over and over, people who receive veganism announce that their skin clears up (skin inflammation, psoriasis, and so forth.), their eyes become more white, their hair gets thicker and more advantageous, their nails become more grounded, their vitality levels soar and their sensitivities clear up. Sound too great to even think about being attempt, isn't that so?

These astounding wellbeing tributes can be ascribed to the high mineral and supplement content found in crisp products of the soil, nuts and seeds, vegetables and beans, verdant greens and entire grain nourishments. The American Dietetic Association inferred that a well-arranged veggie lover or vegetarian diet is without a doubt 'healthfully satisfactory,' and may give various medical advantages and treat or counteract certain infections. Truly, a 'well-arranged' veggie lover diet will give you a liberal measure of fundamental nutrients and minerals, so without a doubt, one's wellbeing will undoubtedly improve.

The veggie lover's way of life is both fulfilling and testing simultaneously. Those new to the veggie lover diet ought to have an intensive comprehension and information on this way of life all together make progress to turning out to be vegetarian as simple as could reasonably be expected. This will guarantee that you will know precisely what's in store, and will assist you with coping with and see any difficulties that may emerge. The accompanying 3 hints are particularly for the apprentice vegetarian. They will assist you in understanding how to begin a veggie-lover diet effectively as it were, the means by which to guarantee going great!

Tip # 1 - Know in Advance the Rewards and Challenges

The compensating part of the vegetarian diet includes astounding wellbeing and mental benefits including weight reduction, clear skin, fewer sensitivities, an inversion or decrease of incessant sickness, more slow-maturing procedure, inward harmony and happiness, and capacity to center and focus better.

The difficult perspective includes how loved ones will respond at first and long haul, the longings you will grow (particularly toward the beginning of the eating regimen for the fledgling vegetarian), the test of eating out, introductory detox manifestations, and feeling like somewhat of a weight when individuals must plan distinctive nourishment only for you.

Research others who have gone on the veggie lover diet and see what they have encountered. What did they say was the most testing angle? Did it get simpler for them? Likewise, discover what advantages and rewards they encountered. You will discover in your examination that most society will concur that the prizes by a wide margin exceed any difficulties or impediments experienced on the veggie lover way of life!

Tip # 2 - Find and Collect Great Vegan Recipes

This is one of the most significant hints for progressing to the veggie lover diet. It is basic for each learner veggie lover to begin their new diet completely arranged, i.e., with a lot of extraordinary vegetarian plans. Having a significant measure of plans gathered will guarantee the accompanying:

1. That you can plan something fast and simple when you are feeling worn out or occupied

2. Will spare you the aggravation of chasing for veggie lover plans when you are essentially not in the temperament.

3. At the point when you are longing for a sweet treat, you can go to your formula assortment and heat your sound cake or cut, instead of either going off your eating regimen or eating bundle vegetarian lousy nourishment.

Discover your veggie lover plans online employing sites, websites, you-tube, or by acquiring a vegetarian formula digital book (note: veggie-lover formula digital books contain huge amounts of flavorful plans made by proficient veggie-lover culinary experts). Else, you could buy a veggie-lover formula cookbook at your nearby book shop, yet this is typically the most costly alternative. The decision of where you get your plans is all yours.

Tip # 3 - Let Family, Friends and Co-Workers Know

It is critical to advise dear companions, family, and even collaborators that you are embracing a veggie lover way of life. This will fill in as an insurance for you and will help make your change to the vegetarian diet as calm as could be expected under the circumstances. In what capacity? Here are a couple of situations that you will be protected from:

1. At the point when companions or family come to visit you, they will definitely realize that you are eating just vegetarian nourishment, and will cease from bringing cakes or bread rolls that you can't eat. Truth be told, they will probably have gone to the issue of choosing a veggie-lover treat from the grocery store - just to impart to you!

2. You will be spared from plenty of inquiries and cross-examinations at bistros and cafés since your companions

have just been educated regarding your choice (and likely, to a huge degree, your cross-examination will as of now be over!!!)

3. In get-togethers, end of year festivities, and gatherings, all things considered, the host will guarantee that there is some nourishment there that you can eat. There's nothing more awful than heading off to a gathering and not having the option to eat any of the nourishment (been there, done that. I don't suggest that you put yourself in that circumstance).

Top Five Benefits Of A Plant-Based Diet

1.) Lower Cholesterol

Practicing environmental awareness can significantly bring down the measure of LDL cholesterol in your blood - the terrible kind that can prompt coronary illness and stroke. Maintain a strategic distance from the spread, cut out greasy meats and decide on plant-based nourishments. Dairy and creature items are stacked with Fat and have no fiber. Plant-based nourishments contain no cholesterol at all. That implies vegetarian nourishment is vastly improved for your heart and your wellbeing. It's even been demonstrated by an ongoing report out of St. Michael's Hospital in Toronto, which found that a low-Fat plant-based eating regimen can bring down LDL cholesterol by 28 percent.

2.) Lower Blood Pressure

At the point when you eat greasy meats and dairy items, the consistency of your blood increments, setting more weight on the veins. A plant-based eating routine tops you off with veggies and organic products, which are high in potassium. The higher admission of potassium adjusts blood thickness. This is the reason veggie lovers and vegetarians will, in general, have lower paces of hypertension, "the quiet executioner," as indicated by observational investigations distributed in the Nutrition Review.

3.) Prevent Cancer

High-Fat weight control plans have been connected to higher paces of malignant growth. The Physicians Committee for Responsible Medicine's Cancer Project demonstrated vegans to be 40 percent less inclined to create disease than meat-eaters. The meat will, in general, be high in immersed Fat and low in fiber. Fiber assumes a key job in keeping your stomach related framework perfect and sound, evacuating malignant growth, causing mixes before they can make hurt.

A veggie lover diet and vegetarian diet are high in fiber, low in immersed and trans-Fat s, and normally incorporate more natural products, vegetables, and other disease averting phytochemicals.

4.) Avoid Heart Disease

The American Heart Association says 83 million Americans have some cardiovascular infection, and a considerable lot of the hazard factors, for example, stoutness, are at unsurpassed highs. Be that as it may, you lessen your hazard. Research has discovered that a reasonable, low-Fat, plant-based eating regimen can help lessen cholesterol, add to weight reduction, and lower circulatory strain. All of which lead to heart issues.

5.) Maintain Healthy Weight and Fitness

The individuals who pursue a plant-based, veggie lover or vegan diet, for the most part, expend fewer calories and have lower body loads than the individuals who don't, as per the Mayo Clinic. In any case, a plant-based eating routine doesn't ensure weight reduction. You'll need to keep your admission of desserts and greasy nourishments low, pick entire grains, eat an assortment of foods grown from the ground, and pick without Fat and low-Fat dairy items. Likewise, recollect that cooking Directions checks — steam, bubble, barbecue, or meal as opposed to singing. Your new diet will even give you re-established vitality for physical exercise.

Step by step instructions to Transition to a Plant-Based Diet

Beside basically maintaining a strategic distance from meat, there are approaches to facilitate the change to a fundamentally plant-based eating routine. Increment the measure of grains, and foods are grown from the ground on your plate step by step until the meat is the littlest bit of your supper. An online vegetarian conveyance administration can make the procedure straightforward.

Your Plant-Based Kitchen

I made a rundown for you to utilize when it comes time to stock your kitchen and washroom. It's an extensive rundown yet don't be scared. It's just a rule to give you a thought of the assortment of nourishments overall nourishment plant-based eating regimen.

Start with what you as of now have in your kitchen and washroom. On the off chance that you feel overpowered, start with a couple of various grains, vegetables, herbs and flavors, dried natural products, nuts and seeds, berries and regular foods grown from the ground. After some time, add new things to your menu. Before long, you'll have gathered the greater part of the things beneath or will have at any rate attempted them all.

Rundown Of Nourishments To Stock At Home

Entire Grains, Pasta And Breakfast Oats

Rice (darker, dark, red), quinoa, grain, antiquated wheat assortments spelled and farro, entire wheat, buckwheat, oats, millet, sorghum (without gluten), rye and triticale (crossbreed of wheat and rye), and items made of those entire grains (pasta, lasagne, noodles, oats, flours, breads).

Vegetables

Lentils (red, dark-colored, green, dark), beans (pinto, white, red, dark, kidney, dark peered toward and so forth.), chickpeas. Store them dried and afterward cook them yourself or get them in jars and containers. There are likewise portions of pasta made of lentil flour.

Herbs And Flavors, Dried

This rundown can be exceptionally long, particularly in the event that you like Indian nourishment, yet coming up next is an essential stock to begin: ocean Salt , pepper (dark, red, white, green), bean stew pieces, paprika powder, curry powder or glue, turmeric, garlic powder, onion drops, sound leaves, oregano, rosemary, thyme, basil, savvy, natural vegetable soup powder, caraway seeds, mustard seeds, cinnamon, cardamom, nutmeg, ginger powder.

Herbs And Flavors, New

Basil, parsley, coriander, rosemary, mint, thyme, ginger.
Dried natural products
Prunes, dates, figs, raisins, apricots, goji berries, mulberries.
Crisp (as per season) or solidified berries
Blueberries, dark currants, red currants, fruits, raspberries, strawberries, blackberries.

Nuts And Seeds

Flax seeds, chia seeds, hemp seeds, sesame seeds, sunflower seeds, pumpkin seeds, poppy seeds, Brazil nuts, pecans, cashews, hazelnuts, almonds, destroyed coconut.

Note: ideally eat nuts, seeds, vegetables, and grains that have been splashed and washed. Drenching makes them all the more effectively edible, diminishes or expels phytic corrosive (which lessens mineral ingestion); discharges the Protein inhibitors that store supplements while developing and anticipates untimely germination, and even lift nutrient B content.

Verdant Greens And Plates Of Mixed Greens

Romain lettuce, ice sheet lettuce, arugula, chard, kale, spinach, bokchoy, watercress, radicchio, endive, chicory.

Ocean Growth

Wakame, kombu, nori, agar-agar.

Boring Vegetables

Potatoes, sweet potatoes, parsnips, corn, pumpkin, butternut squash, oak seed squash, green peas, plantains.

Non-Boring Vegetables

Artichokes, beetroot, turnip, carrots, summer squash, chime peppers, tomatoes, leeks, onions, eggplant, cucumber, celery, broccoli, cauliflower, cabbage (green, red, Savoy, Chinese), Brussels grows, green beans, asparagus, okra, radishes, sugar snap peas, mushrooms.

Natural Products

Bananas, apples, pears, oranges, mandarins, avocados, lemons, kiwis, olives, persimmons, mangos, grapefruit, watermelon, melon.

Other

Dietary yeast, cacao powder, carob powder, dim chocolate (in any event 72% cacao substance) or cacao glue, balsamic vinegar.

Useful for those on the move and for uncommon treats

Soy sauce (search for one that has a low sodium content), agave syrup, xylitol, stevia.

Eateries and bistros are decent choices when meeting companions or on the off chance that you simply need to take a break from the kitchen. I know it is difficult to discover places that take into account plant-based entire nourishments, yet it tends to be finished.

When feasting out, settle on a veggie lovers or vegan cafés or eateries that offer some veggie lover things on their menus. Do your examination utilizing Happy Cow (happycow.net).

Check the online menus of new places. On the off chance that you don't perceive any undeniable alternatives for you, at that point, telephone or email the foundation and inquire as to whether it will oblige you.

As of now, at a café? Inquire as to whether they have a veggie-lover menu.

Ensure you indicate you'd like supper with no creature items. Regularly individuals don't have the foggiest idea what veggie lover or plant-based directions and you may wind up with milk or cheddar on your plate.

Try not to be timid about making your very own dish from the fixings off the menu. Most eateries ought to be glad to support you.

Eat before you eat. Once at the café you can arrange a serving of mixed greens or a vegetable soup. Each eatery ought to, at any rate, have one of those two things.

Ethnic cafés are, in every case great alternatives for discovering veggie lovers or vegan dinners. You can, at any rate, get rice and vegetables. Make a point to request that the culinary experts forget about all the Salt and oil, on the off chance that they can.

Serving of mixed greens smorgasbords can be generous. Keep this basic plate rule: ½ non-bland vegetables (crude and cooked), ¼ entire grains and dull vegetables and ¼ Protein (nuts, seeds, vegetables).

On the off chance that there is no entire nourishment dressing at the plate of mixed greens bar, utilize vegetable puree soup, veggie curry or just lemon squeeze. This will assist you in beginning to acknowledge more slender alternatives as well.

A few eateries offer macrobiotic choices, for example, a dish cooked without oils and Salt , simply straightforward and lean entire nourishments. I have had the option to find a few lunch places like this in Barcelona.

On the off chance that you realize that the Protein , some portion of the feast will be unbalanced, solicit them to substitute some from the Protein with vegetables, entire grains, nuts/seeds or avocados.

Pastries look delectable at cafés however it's normally better to skirt the desserts. They are commonly high-Fat and Fat ty bombs. There are special cases, and a few spots offer crude sweets like chia-pudding or nutty treats without included oils and sugar.

Continuously be affable and cordial towards café staff and your sidekicks. In case you're pleasant to them, all things considered, they'll be decent to you. Continuously be appreciative after the staff has obliged your needs.

The above being stated, do roll out an improvement. I generally urge individuals to request without oil, plant-based and entire grain alternatives regardless of whether I realize the spot doesn't offer them. On the off chance that individuals continue requesting these determinations, at that point, who knows? One day the eatery may add them to the menu.

1. Sweet dessert tarte flambée

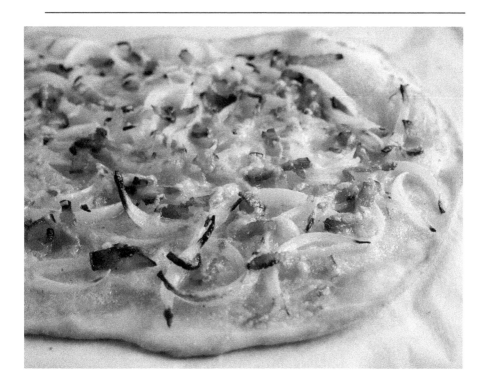

INGREDIENTS

For the dough:
- 1/2 cube of yeast, fresh
- 130 ml of water
- 250 g buckwheat flour
- 2 Tablespoons of sugar
- 1 Tsp salt
- 3 Tablespoons of olive oil

For covering:
- 3 peach

- 3 EL Mandelmus
- 2 EL agave nectar
- 40 g almond, chopped
- mint leaf

PREPARATIONS

1. Crumble the yeast and dissolve in 50 milliliters of lukewarm water. Put the flour in a bowl and press a hollow in the middle. Mix the yeast mixture with the sugar and some flour from the edge of the trough, then let the batter rise for about ten minutes.

2. Add remaining dough INGREDIENTS and knead into a smooth dough that no longer sticks to your hands. If necessary, add a little flour or water for a smooth consistency during kneading. Shape the dough into a ball and leave covered in a warm place for 45 minutes.

3. In the meantime, remove the peach pulp from the core and cut into fine slices.

4. Preheat the oven to 210 degrees (top / bottom heat). Knead the dough again after letting it rise and divide it into two portions. Roll out each dough portion thinly on a piece of baking paper. Brush the flatbread with almond butter. Place peach slices on the dough flat like tiles, drizzle with agave syrup and sprinkle with chopped almonds. Bake

crispy bread on the middle shelf within 15 minutes. Serve half a flame cake sprinkled with mint leaves.

NUTRITION

- calories 470kcal
- carbohydrates 69g
- fat 82g
- Protein 8g

2. No Bake Protein Energy Ball

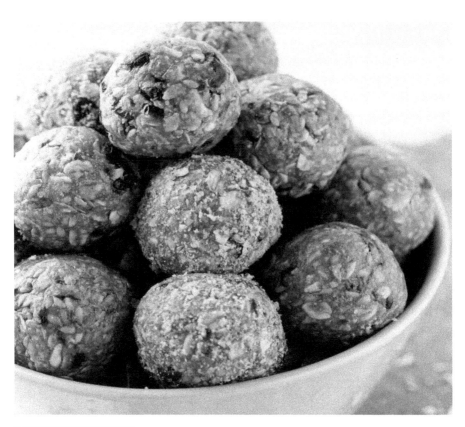

INGREDIENTS

- 2 cups rolled oats , gluten free if needed
- ½ cup pumpkin seeds
- 1 cup hemp seeds
- ½ cup cacao nibs
- 1 cup pecans , any nut works or leave out for nut free
- ½ cups goji berries

- 2 ½ cups dates
- 1 teaspoon vanilla extract
- pinch sea salt
- ½ - ¾ cup water
- ½ cup unsweetened shredded coconut

PREPARATION

1. Place oats, pumpkin seeds, hemp seeds, cacao nibs, and pecans in a large bowl. Place goji berries in a small bowl and fill with warm water. Allow to soak for 5 minutes or until they soften a bit. Once slightly soft, drain water and place berries into the bowl with the rest of the INGREDIENTS.

2. Place dates, vanilla extract, salt and water in a food processor. Mix until partially smooth and partially chunky. This is similar to my date paste recipe but not as smooth and has a tad less water.

3. Put into the bowl with the rest of the INGREDIENTS. Using your hands, mix everything together well until you get a dough like consistency.

NUTRITION

- Calories 225 Carbohydrates 27g Protein 6g Sugar 13g
- Fat 11g

3. Fudge Brownies

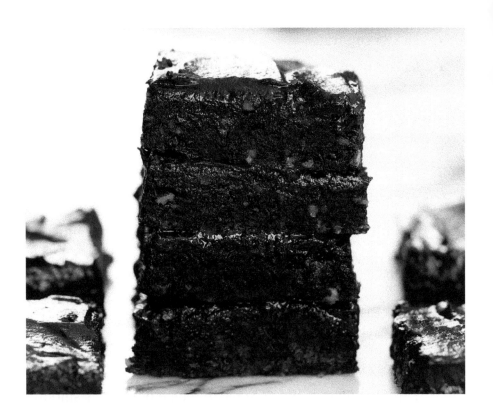

INGREDIENTS

- 3/4 cup gluten-free quick oats
- 1/4 cup water
- 3/4 cup cooked or canned black beans
- 1 medium yellow squash (~200g)
- 1.5 tsp baking powder
- 1/4 cup cocoa powder

- 3/4 cup granulated erythritol
- 1/4 tsp salt
- 1 tsp natural butter flavor
- 1 tsp vanilla extract
- 1/2 tsp liquid stevia

PREPARATIONS

1. Preheat oven to 350F, spray 8×8 baking pan with non-stick cooking spray, an set aside.

2. Add oats to blender and process until flour-like consistency is reached.

3. Add in remaining INGREDIENTS, and blend until smooth.

4. Pour into prepared baking dish, and bake for 30 minutes or until a toothpick inserted into the center comes out clean.

5. Once brownies have cooled, dust with powdered erythritol if desired.

NUTRITION

- Calories 59
- Protein 3g
- Fat 1g
- Sodium 75mg
- Potassium 126mg

4. Pomegranate Masghati Dessert

INGREDIENTS

- 3 cups no-sugar-added pomegranate juice, divided (see Tip)
- 6 tablespoons cornstarch
- ⅓ cup sugar, plus more as needed
- 1 tablespoon rose water (optional)
- ¼ cup pomegranate seeds, plus more for garnish
- Chopped or slivered raw pistachios, for garnish
- Ground dried rose petals, for garnish

PREPARATION

1. Set aside a 9- to 10-inch, 1- to 2-inch-deep serving dish (a regular pie plate works). Whisk 1 cup pomegranate juice with cornstarch in a small bowl until completely smooth, without any lumps; set aside.

2. Combine sugar and the remaining 2 cups pomegranate juice in a medium saucepan. Bring to a simmer (little bubbles start to appear on the sides) over medium-high heat; cook, stirring, until the sugar dissolves, about 5 minutes.

3. Whisk the cornstarch mixture and add it to the saucepan. Reduce the heat to medium-low and start stirring immediately. Continue to stir until it starts to set, 2 to 5

minutes. Don't go anywhere during this process (the cornstarch sets quickly and can burn). You'll know the mixture is ready when it lightly coats the back of a spoon. You don't want it to get too thick, as it will keep setting as it cools. At the very last moment, add rose water (if using) and pomegranate seeds; stir to combine and remove from the heat.

4. Immediately pour the masghati into the serving dish and smooth the top. Set aside to cool to room temperature, then refrigerate, uncovered, to fully set and chill, 6 to 8 hours. Once chilled, garnish with pomegranate seeds, pistachios and rose petals, if desired, and serve cold.

NUTRITION

- 149 calories
- 0.1 g total fat
- 37.2 g carbohydrates
- 0.4 g fiber
- 29 g sugar
- 0.6 g protein

5. Vanilla Cupcakes

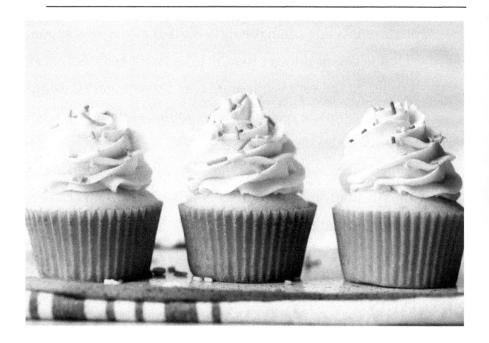

INGREDIENTS

- 1 1/4 cups white whole wheat flour OR 3/4 cup almond meal plus 3/4 cup coconut flour
- 3/4 cup erythritol or sugar
- 1 tsp baking soda
- 1/2 tsp salt
- 1 cup almond milk
- 1 tablespoon vanilla extract
- 1/3 cup applesauce
- 1 tsp distilled white or apple cider vinegar

- 2 tablespoons unsweetened cocoa powder

PREPARATION

1. Preheat oven to 350°F. Line a 12 cup muffin tin with cupcake liners and set aside.
2. In a large bowl, combine the flour, erythritol or sugar, baking soda, and salt. Add in the almond milk, vanilla extract, applesauce, and vinegar until the batter is uniform and no pockets of flour remain. Take care not to over stir. Scoop 1/2 cup of the batter into another bowl and set aside.
3. Evenly distribute the batter into the cupcake liners. The trick to doing this is using an ice cream scoop. It makes the process very neat and keeps the cupcakes the same size so they bake evenly. Bake in the oven at 350°F for about 25 minutes, or until a toothpick inserted into the center comes out clean. Allow to cool before frosting.
4. Meanwhile, add 2 tablespoons of unsweetened cocoa powder and 1 tablespoon almond milk to the reserved 1/2 cup batter and stir until combined. Chill in the fridge until the cupcakes are completely cool. Spread the frosting over the cooled cupcakes and devour.

Nutrition

Calories: 50 cal Fat: 0.5 grams g

6. Macaroons

INGREDIENTS

- 1 cup reduced-fat, unsweetened shredded coconut (such as "Let's Do Organic" brand)
- 1 tbsp flour (such as ww pastry or coconut flour)
- 1/2 cup plus 2 tbsp lite coconut milk
- 3 tbsp pure maple syrup or agave
- pinch uncut stevia (or another tbsp maple/agave)
- 1/4 tsp coconut extract (or vanilla extract)
- tiny bit over 1/16 tsp salt

1. Combine all INGREDIENTS in a tall dish and microwave 2 minutes. (Or cook on the stovetop until it's firm enough to scoop into ball shapes.)
2. Scoop balls onto a cookie tray. (I used a melon baller, but a spoon or ice-cream scoop will work.)
3. Cook at 350 for 8-10 minutes.
4. Let cool before removing from tray.

7. Chocolate Fudge Truffles

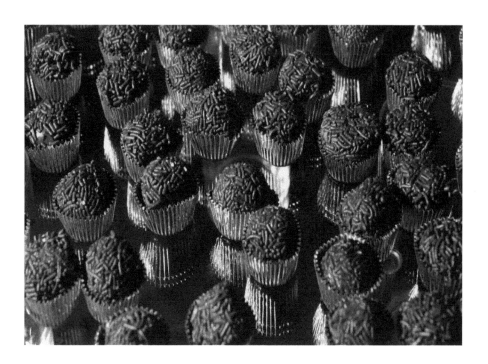

INGREDIENTS

- 1½ cups Homemade Vegan Sweetened Condensed Milk
- 2 tsp Vanilla Creme-Flavored Stevia Extract
- 168g (1¼ cups, lightly packed) Chocolate Brown Rice Protein Powder
- 20g (¼ cup) Unsweetened Dutch Processed Cocoa Powder
- ⅛ tsp Salt

PREPARATION

- In a large bowl, whisk together the condensed milk and stevia extract.
- Add in the protein powder, cocoa powder, and salt. Whisk together until completely combined (mixture should thicken like frosting). Cover and refrigerate the mixture for 5+ hours (mixture should firm up).
- Line a cookie sheet with parchment paper.
- Use a cookie scoop (for the food service peeps, I used the #40 1½ tbs purple disher) to portion the fudge onto the cookie sheet. Refrigerate uncovered for 30 minutes to an hour.
- Roll the scoops between your palms to form balls, then place back in the fridge for another 30 minutes to an hour. Serve and enjoy!

Nutrition
- Calories 100
- Carbohydrates 4g
- protein 12g
- Fat 5g
- Sugar 0.5g

8. Chocolate Avocado Cookies

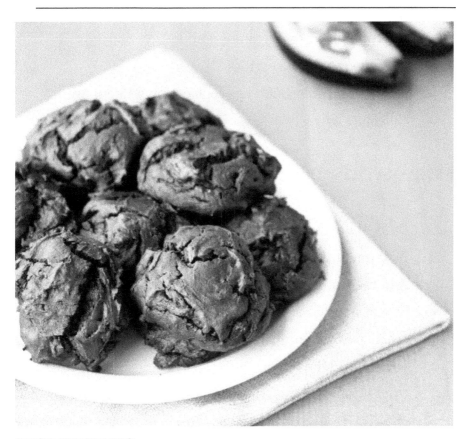

INGREDIENTS

- 2 ¼ cup white whole wheat flour OR 2 3/4 cup almond meal plus 1/4 cup coconut flour
- 1/2 teaspoon salt
- 1 teaspoon baking soda
- 1/2 cup granulated sugar or erythritol

- 1/2 cup brown sugar OR 1/2 cup erythritol plus 1 teaspoon of molasses
- 1/2 cup unsweetened cocoa powder
- 1/4 cup mashed avocado
- 1/4 cup unsweetened almond milk
- 2 teaspoons vanilla extract
- 2 eggs or 1 Tablespoon egg replacer plus ¼ cup water
- chocolate chips

PREPARATION

1. Preheat oven to 350°F. Line a baking sheet with parchment paper or a silicone mat and set aside.
2. Add the flour, salt, baking soda, cane sugar or erythritol, brown sugar or erythritol plus molasses, and unsweetened cocoa powder into the bowl of stand mixer. Alternately, you can add the INGREDIENTS to a large mixing bowl and stir by hand. Using the paddle attachment, stir the dry INGREDIENTS on low speed. Add in the mashed avocado, unsweetened almond milk, vanilla extract, and eggs or egg replacer and continue to stir until combined but not overworked. The dough will be a bit crumbly, but that's okay. Just use your hands to squish it all together. Stir in the chocolate by hand.
3. Using a 1/2 tablespoon measure, scoop the dough into balls and place on the baking sheet two inches apart. Press

down into cookie shapes. Bake in the oven at 350°F for about 12 minutes. Let cool on wire racks. Stored in a ziplock bag in the refrigerator, these cookies should last at least a week. Devour.

NUTRITION

- Calories: 30 cal
- Fat: 0.5 grams g

9. Avocado Chocolate Mousse

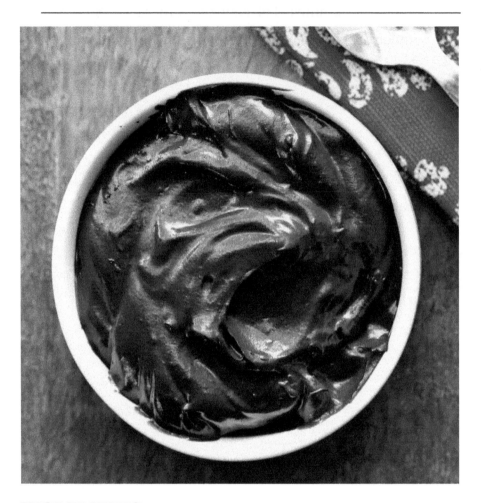

INGREDIENTS

- 1¼ cups unsweetened almond milk or canned coconut milk
- 1 pound dairy-free dark chocolate, preferably 60% cacao, coarsely chopped
- 4 small ripe avocados—pitted, peeled and chopped

- ¼ cup agave syrup
- 1 tablespoon finely grated orange zest
- 2 tablespoons puffed quinoa
- 2 teaspoons Maldon sea salt
- 2 teaspoons Aleppo pepper flakes
- 1 tablespoon extra-virgin olive oil

PREPARATION

1. In a small saucepan, heat the almond or coconut milk over medium-high heat until it registers 175°F on an instant-read thermometer. Remove from the heat and stir in the chopped chocolate until melted; let cool to room temperature.

2. In the bowl of a blender, combine the avocados, agave, orange zest and cooled chocolate mixture; blend on high speed until smooth.

3. To serve, divide the mousse among four bowls. Sprinkle evenly with the puffed quinoa, sea salt and Aleppo pepper, and drizzle with the olive oil.

NUTRITION

- 596 calories
- 42g fat
- 92g carbs
- 26g protein
- 12g sugars

10.   Golden Mylk Cheesecak

INGREDIENTS

Almond Crust

- 1 tablespoon flax meal
- 1½ cups whole almonds
- 3 tablespoons coconut oil
- 2 tablespoons agave

Golden Milk Cheesecake Filling

- 16 ounces vegan cream cheese, at room temperature
- 1½ cups vegan powdered sugar
- ¾ cup coconut milk
- 1 teaspoon ground turmeric, plus more for finishing
- ½ teaspoon ground ginger
- ½ teaspoon ground cinnamon
- Pinch black pepper
- Toasted coconut flakes, for finishing

PREPARATION

1. **MAKE THE ALMOND CRUST:** Preheat the oven to 375°F. Place a 9-inch springform pan on a baking sheet.

2. In a medium bowl, mix together 3 tablespoons water and the flax meal.

3. In the bowl of a food processor, pulse the almonds until they're finely chopped. Transfer to the bowl with the flax mixture and mix in the coconut oil, agave and egg white until well combined.

4. Press the mixture into the base and halfway up the sides of the springform pan. Bake until the crust is lightly golden, 12 to 14 minutes. Cool completely.

5. MAKE THE GOLDEN MYLK CHEESECAKE FILLING: Wipe out the bowl of the food processor. Add the cream cheese, vegan powdered sugar, coconut milk, turmeric, ginger, cinnamon and black pepper to the food processor and puree until smooth.

6. Pour the filling into the crust and transfer to the refrigerator. Chill until the filling is set, 2 to 3 hours. Leave the cheesecake chilled until you're ready to serve.

7. To serve, dust with turmeric and serve with toasted coconut flakes.

NUTRITION

Almond Crust
- 172 calories 15g fat 8g carbs 5g protein 4g sugars

Golden Mylk Cheesecake Filling
- 236 calories 17g fat 23g carbs 3g protein 19g sugars

11.   Peanut Butter Mudslide Ice Cream

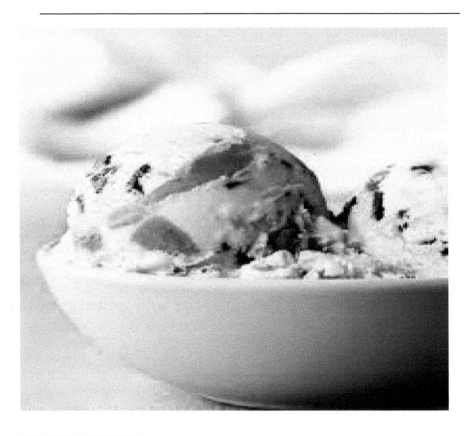

INGREDIENTS

-
- 1 cup dark chocolate chips
- 3 cans coconut cream, divided
- 1/4 cup peanut butter
- 1/2 cup granulated sugar
- 2 teaspoons vanilla extract

- 1/4 teaspoon salt
- 1/4 cup graham cracker crumbs

PREPARATION

1. In a blender, combine all but 1/2 cup of the coconut cream with peanut butter, sugar, vanilla extract, and salt until smooth. Remove and place into fridge for at least 2 hours.

2.

3. Once chilled, begin to assemble your ice cream. In a small saucepan, heat 1/2 cup of the coconut cream over low heat until scalding. Remove from heat, add in chocolate chips, and allow to sit for 5 minutes. After 5 minutes, stir to combine. Chocolate chips should be fully melted by this point! Allow to cool to room temperature while you churn your ice cream base.

4. Place coconut cream mixture into an ice cream maker and churn according to manufacturers PREPARATION.

5. Scoop half of ice cream into freezer-safe container, then spoon in half of ganache mixture and half of graham cracker crumbs. Top with remaining half of ice cream and remaining half of ganache and graham cracker crumbs. Swirl with a knife, then place in freezer for at least 8 hours, preferably overnight.

12. Lemon Cake

INGREDIENTS

Bark

- 2½ cups of nuts
- 1 cup of boneless dates
- 2 tablespoons of maple syrup or agave

To Fill

- 3 cups of prepared cauliflower rice (without salt and pepper)
- 3 avocados, halved and boneless
- 1½ cups of crushed pineapple
- ¾ cup of maple syrup or agave

Zest and juice of 1 lemon

- ½ teaspoon of pure vanilla extract
- ½ teaspoon of lemon extract
- A pinch of cinnamon

Additive

- 1½ cups of natural coconut yogurt (or other milk-free yogurt)
- 1 teaspoon of pure vanilla extract
- 3 tablespoons of maple syrup or agave

PREPARATION

1. Place the outer ring of a 9-inch springform pan on a parchment-lined baking sheet.

2. **MAKE THE CRUST:** In the bowl of a food processor, pulse the pecans until they are finely ground. Add the dates and maple syrup, and pulse until the mixture comes together, about 1 minute.

3. Transfer the mixture to the prepared springform ring and press it into an even layer. Wipe out the bowl of the food processor.

4. **MAKE THE FILLING:** In the food processor, combine the cauliflower rice with the avocados, pineapple, maple syrup, lemon zest and lemon juice. Process until the mixture is very smooth.

5. Add the vanilla extract, lemon extract and cinnamon; pulse to combine. Pour the mixture into the prepared pan on top of the crust. Transfer to the freezer and freeze until very firm (at least 5 hours and up to overnight).

6. Remove the cake from the freezer and let rest at room temperature for 15 to 20 minutes. Remove the outer ring from the cake.

7. **MAKE THE TOPPING:** In a medium bowl, whisk the yogurt with the vanilla extract and maple syrup to combine. Pour onto the cake and spread into an even layer.

13.   Brownies

INGREDIENTS

- 2 cups tightly packed dates, pitted
- 1/4 cup warm water
- 1/2 cup salted peanut butter* (if unsalted, add a healthy pinch of salt to the batter)
- 2 Tbsp melted coconut oil* (if avoiding coconut oil, see notes)
- 1/3 cup cacao or unsweetened cocoa powder
- 1/3 cup dairy-free dark chocolate chips (*optional* // we like Enjoy Life)
- 1/2 cup roughly chopped raw walnuts (*optional* // or other nut of choice)

PREPARATION

1. Preheat oven to 350 degrees F (176 C) and line a standard loaf pan (or similar size pan) with parchment paper. Set aside.
2. Add dates to food processor and blend until small bits or a ball forms. If your food processor has a difficult time processing the dates, ensure there are no pits in the dates *and* that your dates are fresh and sticky. If too dry they can have a difficult time blending. (It may also be an issue of food processor strength if it has a hard time blending.)

3. Once blended, separate the dates into chunks using a spoon. Then add hot water and blend until a sticky date paste forms. Scrape down sides as needed.

4. Add peanut butter, coconut oil, and cacao powder and pulse until a sticky batter forms. It should be tacky and thick (scrape down sides as needed). Lastly add chocolate chips and walnuts (optional) and pulse to incorporate.

5. Transfer batter to lined loaf pan and spread into an even layer. For a smooth top, lay some parchment paper on top and use a flat-bottomed object (like a drinking glass) to press into an even layer.

6. Bake on the center rack for 15 minutes - the edges should be slightly dry. Remove from oven and let cool in the pan for 10 minutes. Then carefully lift out of the pan using the edges of the parchment paper and let cool on a plate or cooling rack for at least 20 minutes before slicing. The longer they cool, the firmer they will become.

7. Enjoy warm or cooled. Store leftovers covered at room temperature up to 3 days, in the refrigerator up to 5-6 days, or in the freezer up to 1 month (let thaw before enjoying).

NUTRITION

- Calories: 215 Fat: 8.1g Carbohydrates: 36.7g Fiber: 3.9g Sugar: 30.4g Protein: 3.6g

14.　　Sea Salt Butterscotch Tart

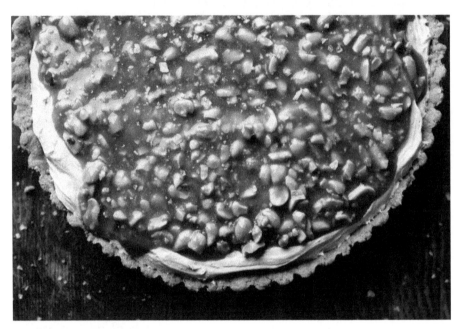

INGREDIENTS

Shortbread Crust

- ½ cup granulated sugar
- ¼ cup virgin coconut oil, at room temperature, or softened butter
- 1 teaspoon pure vanilla extract
- 2 cups almond meal flour
- ½ teaspoon salt

Filling

- ⅔ cup packed light brown sugar or coconut sugar

- ⅔ cup canned coconut cream
- ½ cup coconut oil or butter
- 1 teaspoon kosher salt
- Flaked sea salt, as needed
- 1 Granny Smith apple, sliced (optional)

PREPARATION

1. Preheat the oven to 375 ° F and place a 9-inch or 4-by-14-inch cake pan nearby.

2. PREPARE THE BARK: In a bowl with a hand mixer or a food processor with a paddle, stir the granulated sugar, coconut oil and vanilla until they are foamy. Mix almond flour and salt. Then press the mixture evenly over the bottom and sides of the cake pan.

3. Place the entire cake pan in the freezer for 10 minutes to harden, then bake in the oven until the edge is golden and the center is crispy (15 minutes). Remove from the oven and let cool.

4. MAKE THE FILLING: Mix the brown sugar, coconut cream, coconut oil and salt in a saucepan. Bring to the boil and cook over medium heat for about 25 minutes. Drink a cup of ice water nearby. Dip the tip of a fork in the boiling sugar and then in the ice water; If the sugar sticks between the forks without dissolving, the filling is done. Pour it into the cooled crust, sprinkle it with sea salt, place the apple slices on it as desired and let it cool and harden before cutting and serving.

NUTRITION

- 431 calories 33g fat 32g carbs 6g protein 27g sugars

15. Vegetarian Chocolate-Covered Digestive Biscuits

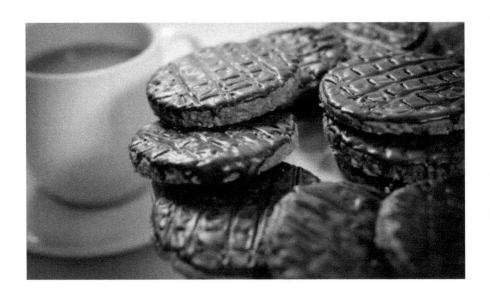

INGREDIENTS

- 1 cup whole wheat plain flour
- 3/4 cup plain flour
- 3 tablespoons caster sugar
- 1/2 teaspoon baking powder
- 1/4 teaspoon Salt
- 1/3 cup vegan butter
- 1-2 tablespoons soy milk or preferred non-dairy milk

For the Chocolate Topping:

- 1/3 cup vegan chocolate

- 1 tablespoon coconut oil

DIRECTIONS

1. Preheat oven to 350°F fan-forced and line two baking trays with grease proof paper.
2. In a medium sized mixing bowl, mix together the flours, sugar, baking powder and Salt . Rub in the butter using your fingertips. Using your hands, mix in 1 tablespoon of the milk at a time, until it creates a soft dough. I only needed 1 1/2 tablespoons.
3. Form the dough into a ball and place on an extra piece of grease proof paper. Roll it out to an even 1/8-inch thick. Using a 2 and 1/2-inch cookie cutter, cut out as many circles as you can, placing them 1-inch apart on the baking trays. Reroll the dough scraps and continue cutting until you have no more dough.
4. Bake in the oven for 20-25 minutes or until the edges are lightly golden. Remove and leave to cool completely on the tray.
5. Melt the chocolate and coconut oil in a double boiler and spread over the tops of the cooled biscuits.
6. Leave to set or enjoy as is.

Nutrition: Per Serving

- Calories: 108
- Carbs : 12g
- Fat : 7g
- Protein : 2g
- Sodium: 29mg
- Sugar: 2g

16. Natively constructed Wheat Thins

INGREDIENTS (12 Crackers)

- 3/4 cup DIY Gluten-Free Flour Blend*
- 2/3 cup almond meal* (or sub gluten-free oat flour*)
- 1/4 tsp baking powder
- 2 Tbsp flaxseed meal
- 1 tsp fresh chopped rosemary
- 1/2 tsp sea Salt
- 1/8 tsp garlic powder (*optional*)
- 3.5 Tbsp neutral oil (i.e. grape seed or avocado oil)
- 3-5 Tbsp cold water

DIRECTIONS

1. Preheat oven to 325 degrees F (165 C) and line 1 large or 2 small baking sheets with parchment paper (adjust number of baking sheets if altering batch size).
2. Add dry ingredients to a food processor or a mixing bowl and process or whisk until thoroughly combine.
3. Then add oil and pulse/use a pastry cutter or fork until crumbly.

4. Add cold water 1 Tbsp at a time, pulsing/stirring until it forms a semi-sticky dough that's moldable with your hands and not crumbly. It shouldn't need more than 5 Tbsp (amount as original recipe is written // adjust if altering batch size).

5. Remove from processor or mixing bowl and form into a loose ball with your hands. Transfer to a clean surface lined with wax or parchment paper. Lay another sheet of parchment paper or wax paper on top and use a rolling pin to roll the dough out into a rectangle slightly less than 1/8th inch thick (see photo).

6. Use a knife, a pizza cutter, or a small cookie cutter to cut the dough into squares (or circles). Makes about 60 squares (amount as original recipe is written // adjust if altering batch size).

7. Transfer the dough (still on the wax paper or parchment) to a baking sheet and pop in the freezer for about 10 minutes to stiffen. This will help them firm up and become easier to transfer to the baking sheet.

8. Once firm, use a spatula to carefully transfer the crackers to the parchment-lined baking sheet(s) in a single layer, making sure they aren't touching to ensure even baking.

9. Bake for 16-22 minutes or until slightly golden brown (be careful not to burn). Remove from oven and let cool.

10. Enjoy immediately. Store leftovers covered at room temp for up to 1 week or in the freezer for 1 month.

Nutrition: Per Serving (1 of 12 five-cracker servings)

- Calories: 101
- Fat : 6.8g
- Saturated Fat : 0.8g
- Sodium: 80mg
- Carbohydrates: 9g
- Fiber: 1.8g
- Protein : 1.8g

17.   Veggie lover Spinach and Artichoke Dip

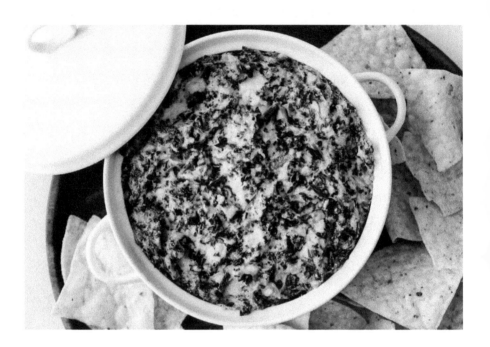

INGREDIENTS

- 13.75 oz artichoke hearts packed in water, drained
- 10 oz frozen spinach, thawed and squeezed
- 1/4 cup chopped shallots
- 1 clove garlic
- 1/2 cup Fat -free Greek yogurt
- 1/2 cup light mayonnaise
- 2/3 cup good quality grated parmesan

- 4 oz shredded part-skim mozzarella cheese
- Salt and fresh pepper to taste
- olive oil spray

DIRECTIONS

1. Preheat oven to 375°F.
1. In a small food processor, coarsely chop the artichoke hearts with the garlic and shallots.
2. Combine all the ingredients in a medium bowl.
3. Place in an oven-proof dish and bake at 375F for 20-25 minutes, until hot and cheese is melted. Serve right away.

Nutrition: Per Serving (1/4 Cup)

- Serving: 1/4 cup, Calories: 73Kcal   Carbohydrates: 3.5g Protein   : 5g   Fat   : 4.5g   Saturated   Fat   : 2g Cholesterol: 10.5mg Sodium: 245mg Fiber: 1g Sugar: 0.5g

18. Za'atar (Thyme-, Sesame-, and Sumac-Spiced) Popcorn

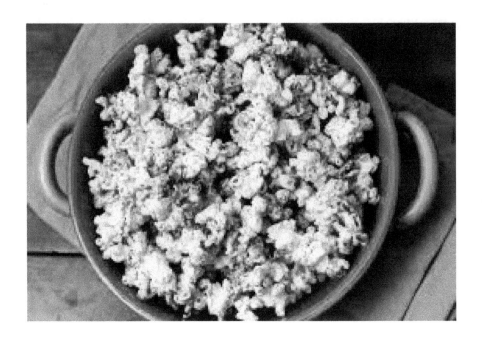

INGREDIENTS

- 8 cups popped popcorn, still hot
- 2 tablespoons extra virgin olive oil
- 1/2 teaspoon Salt (*omit if your za'atar blend already contains Salt)
- 2 tablespoons za'atar
- 1/4 teaspoon freshly ground pepper

DIRECTIONS

Pour oil over hot popcorn, toss to coat. In a small bowl, mix Salt , za'atar, and pepper. Pour mixture over popcorn and toss until well-incorporated.

Notes:
Add 1/2 teaspoon cayenne pepper for a spicy kick
If serving to non-vegans, add freshly grated Parmesan

Nutrition: Per Serving

- 47 Calories per Cup
- 1g sugar
- 2g of Protein

19.   Sweet Potato "Quesadillas"

INGREDIENTS

- 3 small sweet potatoes — *scrubbed but not peeled*
- 1 tablespoon chili powder
- 1 tablespoon cinnamon
- 1 teaspoon cumin
- 1 teaspoon smoked paprika
- 1/2 teaspoon kosher Salt — *divided*
- 1/2 teaspoon ground chipotle chili pepper
- 2 teaspoons extra virgin olive oil
- 1 medium yellow onion — *diced*
- 1 large green bell pepper — *cored and diced*
- 2 cloves minced garlic
- 1 can reduced sodium black beans — *(15 ounces) rinsed and drained*
- 6 medium-sized 100% whole wheat flour tortillas
- 1 1/4 cups freshly grated sharp shredded cheddar cheese

DIRECTIONS

1. Cut potatoes into 1-inch chunks. Place in a large saucepan, cover with water, then bring to a boil. Continue boiling until the potato chunks are fork tender, about 8 minutes. Remove pot from heat, drain the potatoes, then

return the potatoes to the pot and mash. Stir in the chili powder, cinnamon, cumin, smoked paprika, 1/4 teaspoon kosher Salt , and chipotle chili pepper until incorporated. Set aside.

2. Meanwhile, heat the olive oil in a large skillet. Add the onions and peppers and sauté until beginning to soften, about 3 minutes. Add the garlic and remaining 1/4 teaspoon Salt . Continue to sauté until onions are translucent, about 5 minutes more. Stir the sautéed vegetables into sweet potato mash. Stir in black beans until all ingredients are evenly distributed.

3. Heat a large skillet over medium heat, then lightly coat with cooking spray. Place a single tortilla in skillet, then spoon a heaping 1/2 cup of filling onto half of the tortilla and sprinkle with 3 tablespoons of shredded cheese. Fold the empty half of tortilla over the top. Let cook until the bottom of the tortilla is browned and lightly crispy (about 1-2 minutes), then flip and brown the other side. Serve immediately with any desired toppings.

Nutrition: Per Serving

- *Amount per serving (1 quesadilla without extra toppings)* Calories: 364   Fat : 13g   Saturated Fat : 5g   Cholesterol: 25mg   Sodium: 716mg   Carbohydrates: 52g   Fiber: 10g Sugar: 9g Protein : 15g

20.   Stove Roasted Tomato
Bruschetta

INGREDIENTS

- 20 cherry tomatoes
- 1/2 teaspoon coconut oil
- 1 dash Salt , or more, to taste
- 1/4 teaspoon balsamic vinegar
- 1 pinch garlic powder
- 2 large slices white bread, homemade or store bought (I used gluten-free)
- 1/2 teaspoon fresh basil, chopped

DIRECTIONS

1. Wash and halve the cherry tomatoes.
2. Toss them in a pan with the coconut oil--keep on medium to high heat.
3. Start by adding Salt , balsamic vinegar, and garlic powder.
4. Keep it on high heat and stir occasionally.
5. In the meantime, toast the white bread slices in a pan, on an electric griller, or in the oven.

6. Once the tomatoes lose most of their water and look good to you, put them on the white bread slices and top with fresh basil.
7. They are best enjoyed fresh and warm, otherwise the bread gets soggy

Nutrition: Per Serving

- Calories: 106Kcal
- Carbohydrates: 19g
- Protein : 3g
- Fat : 1g
- Saturated Fat : 1g
- Sodium: 161mg
- Potassium: 399mg
- Fiber: 1g
- Sugar: 5g

21. Stove Dried Grapes

INGREDIENTS

- 3 large bunches seedless grapes, preferably mixed colors, stemmed
- Vegetable or canola oil, for greasing

DIRECTIONS

1 . Preheat oven to 225°F (110°C). Very lightly grease 2 rimmed baking sheets with oil, then scatter grapes all over. Bake, checking periodically for doneness, until grapes are nicely shriveled and semi-dried but still slightly plump, about 4 hours (see note). (The exact time will depend on your grapes, your oven, and your preferred degree of dryness.) Let cool. Use a thin metal spatula to free any grapes that are stuck to the baking sheet.

2. The dried grapes can be refrigerated in a sealed container for about 3 weeks. (How long they keep will also depend on their degree of dryness; drier grapes will keep longer.)

Nutrition: Per Serving
One small box (1.5 ounces),129 calories, 1.6g fiber

22. Avocado Toast With Radishes, Baby Peas, and Fresh Herbs

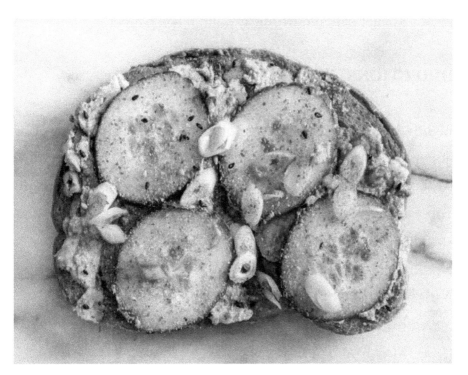

INGREDIENTS

- 1 slice country or sandwich bread, approximately 1/2 inch thick
- Small handful baby peas (see note), or enough to lightly cover surface of bread
- Extra-virgin olive oil
- 1/2 medium pitted and peeled Hass avocado

- 6 thin slices radish from 1 to 2 radishes, or enough to cover surface of bread
- Freshly squeezed lemon juice to taste, from 1/2 lemon
- Finely chopped basil leaves, for garnish
- Kosher salt and freshly ground black pepper

DIRECTIONS

Lightly brush bread with olive oil and toast to desired level of doneness. Top with avocado and mash with a fork to cover entire surface. Add peas, pressing gently to anchor them in avocado. Top with radish slices. Squeeze lemon juice over surface and sprinkle with basil, salt, and pepper. Serve.

Nutrition: Per Serving
- KCal 451
- KCal from Fat 216
- Fat 24g
- Carbohydrates 43g
- Fiber 17g
- Sugar 3g
- Protein 14g

23.   The Best Applesauce

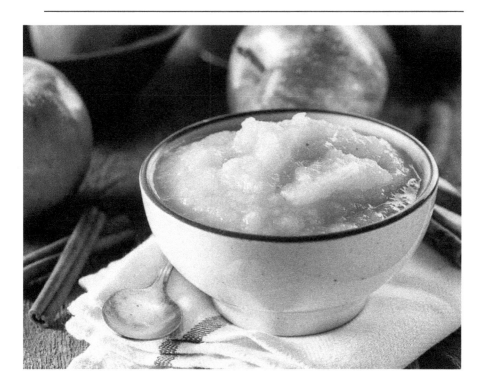

INGREDIENTS

- BASIC APPLESAUCE
- 5 pounds apples combination   of   McIntosh,   Golden Delicious, Granny Smith, Fuji, and Jonathan
- 1 cup water
- 2 tablespoons lemon juice
- 1 3-inch cinnamon stick
- OPTIONAL ADD INS
- 1/2 cup brown sugar

- 2 tablespoons butter
- 1/2 teaspoon ground cinnamon
- 1/2 teaspoon vanilla extract

DIRECTIONS

BASIC APPLESAUCE

Peel, core, and slice apples into small chunks. Transfer to a large saucepan or pot.

Add in water, lemon juice, and cinnamon stick. Bring to a boil over high heat and then reduce the heat to low. Cover and let simmer 20-30 minutes until apples are soft.

Puree using a blender, food processor, or immersion blender for a smoother applesauce.

OPTIONAL ADD INS

For sweetened applesauce, return pureed applesauce to pan. Stir in brown sugar and continue to cook, uncovered, until the applesauce thickens, about 10 minutes.

For a more flavorful, dessert type applesauce, stir in butter, ground cinnamon, and vanilla extract until butter is melted.

SERVING AND STORAGE

Serve warm or cold, or freeze or can using proper canning procedures for later use. Applesauce will stay good refrigerated in an airtight container for up to 2 weeks.

Nutrition: Per Serving

- Calories: 335kcal
- Carbohydrates: 74g
- Protein: 1g
- Fat: 6g
- Saturated Fat: 3g
- Cholesterol: 15mg

24. Simple Vegan Crispy Tofu Spring Rolls with Peanut-Tamarind Dipping Sauce

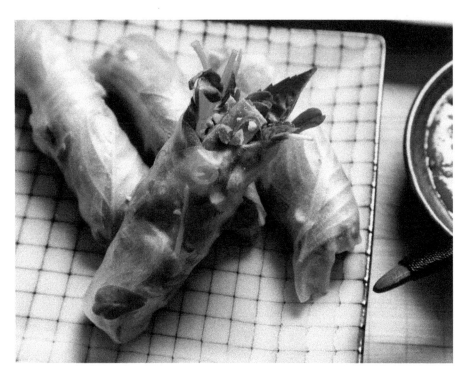

INGREDIENTS

- 1 (14-ounce; 400g) block firm (non-silken) tofu, cut into matchsticks approximately 2 inches long and 1/2 inch square
- 3 tablespoons (45ml) vegetable oil
- 1 recipe Peanut-Tamarind Dipping Sauce

- 1 large carrot, peeled and cut into a fine julienne
- 4 ounces pea greens
- 2 cups mixed picked fresh herbs, such as cilantro, mint, and Thai basil
- Chopped toasted peanuts
- Finely sliced Thai bird or serrano chili peppers
- 20 dried spring roll rice paper wrappers

DIRECTIONS

1. Place tofu in a large colander and set in the sink. Pour 1 quart boiling water over tofu and let rest for 1 minute. Transfer to a paper towel–lined tray and press dry. Heat vegetable oil in a large nonstick or cast iron skillet over medium-low heat until shimmering. Add tofu and cook, turning occasionally, until golden brown and crisp on all surfaces, about 10 minutes total. Transfer to a paper towel–lined plate to drain.

2. Transfer drained tofu to a large bowl and add 5 tablespoons peanut-tamarind sauce. Toss to coat tofu.

3. Transfer tofu, carrots, greens, herbs, peanuts, peppers, and remaining dipping sauce to serving platters. Serve with rice paper wrappers and a bowl of warm water. To eat, dip a rice paper wrapper in warm water until moist on all surfaces, then transfer to your plate. Place a small amount of desired fillings in the center. Roll the front edge of the wrapper over the filling away from you, then

fold the right side over toward the center. Continue rolling until a tight roll with one open end has formed. Dip spring roll in dipping sauce as you eat.

25.   Sparkling Strawberry Mint-Infused Water

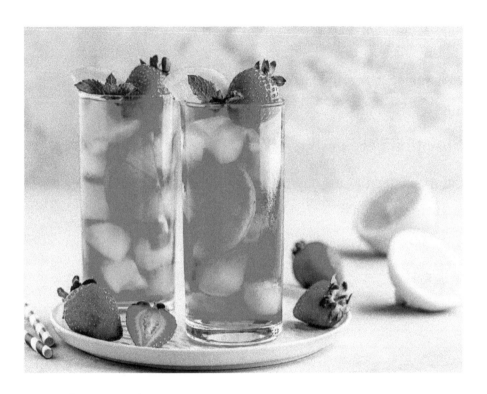

Prep Time: 10 minutes

Serves: 4

Ingredients:

- 3 1/2 cup of fresh lemon juice
- 2 teaspoon of large fresh mint leaves
- 4 mint sprigs
- 4 large fresh strawberries, stemmed

- Sparkling water

Instructions:

1. Add the strawberries, lemon juice and the rest of the ingredients except the fresh mint in a blender and blend in short bursts until smooth.

2. Transfer to serving glasses and serve with a sprig of fresh mint.

Nutrition per Serving

Calories: 5kcal | Carbohydrates: 2g | Protein: 8g | Fiber: 4g | Sugar: 1.4g |15mg

26.   Spicy Tofu Quesadillas

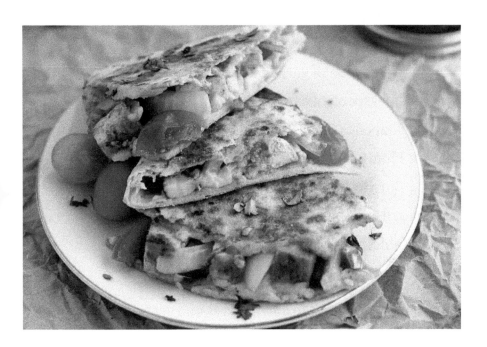

Prep Time: 10 minutes

Cook Time: 20 minutes

Serves: 5

Ingredients:

- 1 Lime, juiced
- 14 oz of firm tofu
- 1/2 teaspoon of salt
- 1 teaspoon of paprika
- 1/2 teaspoon of oregano

- 2 Scallions, sliced thinly
- 1 teaspoon of ground cumin
- 1 tablespoon of chili powder
- 1/4 teaspoon of black pepper
- 1/2 teaspoon of garlic powder
- 1/4 teaspoon of cayenne pepper
- 2 jalapeños, seeded and minced
- 2 Plum Tomatoes, halved and deseeded
- 4 Burrito-Sized flour tortillas
- 2 1/2 cups of shredded cheddar Cheese
- 1 tablespoon of canola oil

Instructions:

1. First, chop tomatoes to small pieces and set aside.

2. Wrap tofu in a paper towel and press until excess water is drained off it. Chop into half inch cubes and set aside.

3. Next, combine the paprika, cumin, chili powder, oregano, garlic powder, salt and pepper to a small bowl and whisk until well combined.

4. Add tofu, half of the lime juice to the spice mixture and stir until well coated.

5. Heat a tablespoon of oil in a non stick skillet over medium heat, add tofu cubes and cook for 10 minutes. Stir regularly so it does not stick, remove from heat and set aside.

6. Place a tortilla on a clean flat surface, on one half, place 1/2 cup of shredded cheese, 1 tablespoon of scallions, 1/4 of the tofu cubes, 1/4 cups of tomatoes and 1 tablespoon of jalapeno.

7. Fold the tortilla and place on a skillet set over low heat and cook until both sides are crisp and lightly browned.

Nutrition per Serving

Calories: 216kcal | Carbohydrates: 2g | Protein: 22g | Fiber: 4g | Sugar: 1.4g |15mg | Total Fat 27g |

27.   Cranberry Apple Cider

12 - Servings

Ingredients:

- Whole cranberries, 2 cups
- Cinnamon sticks, 10
- Nutmeg, 2 teaspoons
- Ground cinnamon, 2 teaspoons
- Whole allspice, 15 to 20
- Whole cloves, 15 to 20
- Cranberry juice, 4 cups
- Apple cider, 8 cups

Instructions:

1.Place all of the ingredients in a slow cooker. Stir to combine.

2.Place lid on slow cooker. Set it to the low setting and allow to cook six hours or until heated through

3.Ladle into mugs and enjoy warm.

Nutrition Facts: Calories: 144.6 Fats: 1 gram Proteins: 6.5 grams Carbohydrates: 30.3 gram

28.   Grilled Avocado in Curry Sauce

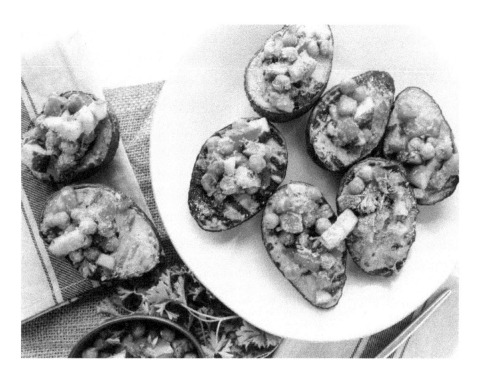

Serves: 2

Preparation time: 15 minutes

Cooking time: 25-30 minutes

Ingredients:

- 1 large avocado, chopped
- ¼ cup water
- 1 tbsp curry, ground
- 2 tbsp olive oil

- 1 tsp soy sauce
- 1 tsp fresh parsley, finely chopped
- ¼ tsp red pepper flakes
- ¼ tsp sea salt

Preparation:

1. Peel the avocado and cut lengthwise in half. Remove the pit and cut the remaining avocado into small chunks. Set aside.
2. Heat up the olive oil in a large saucepan over a medium-high temperature.
3. In a small bowl, combine ground curry, soy sauce, parsley, red pepper and sea salt.
4. Add water and cook for about 5 minutes, stirring occasionally.
5. Add chopped avocado, stir well and cook for 3 more minutes, or until all the liquid evaporates.
6. Turn off the heat and cover. Let it stand for about 15-20 minutes before serving.

Nutrition information per serving: Calories: 338, Protein: 2.5g, Total Carbs: 10.8g, Dietary Fibers: 7.9g, Total Fat: 34.1g

29.   Banana Peanut Butter Ice Cream

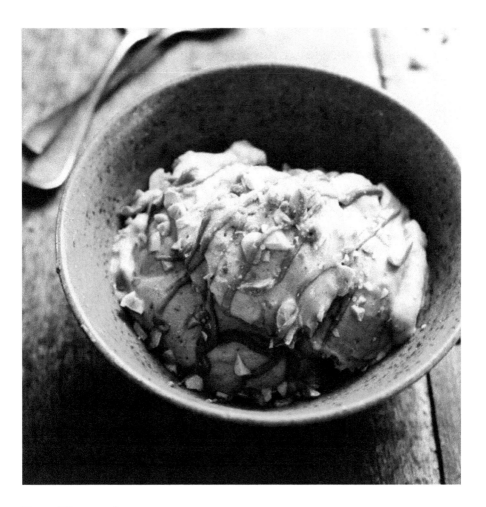

Prep Time: 2 hours

Total Time: 2 hours

Servings: 4

Ingredients:

- 4 large ripe bananas
- 2 tablespoons peanut butter

Preparation:

1. Peel bananas, slice into discs and freeze 2 hours on a large plate.

2. Process until smooth. Add the peanut butter and process as well. Add 2 tablespoons of milk, if desired, for a more creamy consistency.

3. Make Ahead: freeze or refrigerate for up to a week.

Nutrition Per Serving Calories: 152kcal | Fat: 4g |Carbs: 29g | Protein: 3g| Fiber4g|- Sodium: 38mg |

30. Hummus Dip

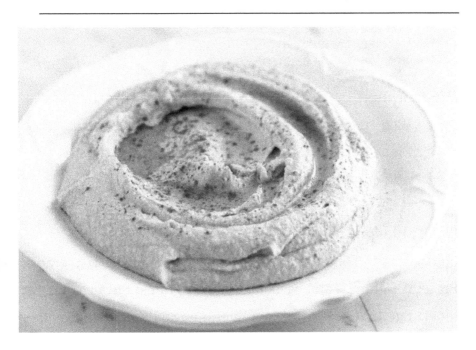

Ingredients

- 2 (15-ounce) cans chickpeas, drained and rinsed
- 1/2 cup extra-virgin olive oil, or more as needed, plus more for garnish
- 1/2 lemon, juiced
- 2 tablespoons roughly chopped fresh parsley leaves, plus more for garnish
- 2 cloves garlic, peeled
- 1 1/2 teaspoon salt
- 1/2 teaspoon dark Asian sesame oil
- 1/2 to 1 teaspoon ground cumin

- 12 to 15 grinds black pepper
- 1/4 cup water
- Paprika, for garnish

Directions

1. Blend together everything but parsley and paprika.
2. Blend until smooth on a low setting.
3. Add garnish. Chill

Per Tablespoon

Calories: 57; Total Fat: 4 grams; Saturated Fat: 0.5 grams; Protein: 1 gram; Total carbohydrates: 5 grams; Sugar: 0 grams; Fiber: 1 gram; Cholesterol: 0 milligrams; Sodium: 96 milligrams

31.   Sweet and spicy snack mix

Serves 12

Ingredients

- 2 cans (15 ounces each) garbanzos, rinsed, drained and patted dry
- 2 cups Wheat Chex cereal
- 1 cup dried pineapple chunks
- 1 cup raisins
- 2 tablespoons honey
- 2 tablespoons reduced-sodium Worcestershire sauce
- 1 teaspoon garlic powder
- 1/2 teaspoon chili powder

Directions

1. Turn on oven to 350. Grease a large baking sheet with low fat oil or cooking spray.
2. Put garbanzo beans in pan and cook until brown or for about 10 minutes.
3. Put beans on cooking sheet. Add cooking spray. Bake until crisp or for about twenty minutes.
4. Spray roasting pan with cooking spray. Add cereal, raisins, and pineapple. Add beans and stir.
5. In a large glass bowl add honey, spices, and Worcestershire sauce. Mix. Back an additional 15 minutes. Remove and cool.

Nutritional analysis per serving

Serving size: 1/2 cup

Calories 154 Sodium 192 mg Total fat trace Total carbohydrates 36 g Saturated fat trace Dietary fiber 3 g Monounsaturated fat trace Protein 3 g Cholesterol 0 mg

32.   Creamy Rice Pudding with Blueberry Compote

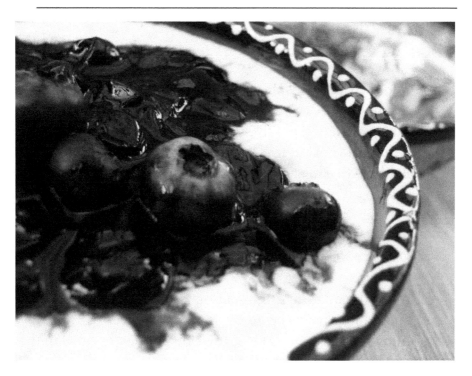

Prep Time: Time: 1 Hour

Serves: 8 – 10

Ingredients:

- Rice Pudding:
- 1 ½ cup Basmati Rice – brown, organic
- 2 ½ cups Water
- 1 pinch Salt
- 4 cups Rice Milk
- ½ cup Demerara sugar
- 2 tbsp. Potato Starch

- Cinnamon powder – to taste
- For the Blueberry Compote:
- 3 cups fresh, organic Blueberries
- ½ cup Sugar
- ¼ cup Water

Directions:

1. Add the rice and water to a medium saucepan and bring to a boil.
2. Add the salt and gently stir the contents. Once boiled, reduce the heat to low, and simmer the rice.
3. Fold the rice in gently until all the water is fully absorbed.
4. Add to this, the brown sugar and 2 pinches of cinnamon powder and mix. Add the rice milk and continue to cook for about 10 minutes.
5. Dissolve the potato starch in a few tablespoon of water and add to the rice mix.
6. Allow the mixture to simmer on low heat until it thickens and remove from the heat.
7. Allow to cool, and transfer to a bowl. Place the bowl in the fridge and allow it to cool.
8. In a small saucepan on medium heat, crush the blueberries to a small pot and add the sugar and water.
9. Bring to boil and allow it to simmer. Remove from the heat after a minute or two.
10. Once chilled, serve with the warm Blueberry compote.

33. Raspberry Apple Crumble

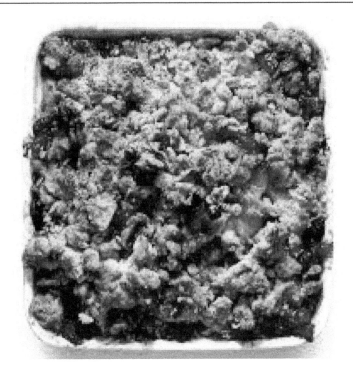

Prep Time:: 1 Hour 15 minutes

Serves: 4-6

Ingredients:

- 6 large cooking Apples – thinly sliced
- 1 cup Raspberries
- 2.5 cups Apple Juice
- 2.5 cups Rolled Oats
- ¼ cup Butter (or) Margarine
- 3 tbsp. Brown Sugar (Demerara)
- 1.5 tsp Cinnamon powder
- 1.5 tbsp. Clove powder

Directions:

1. Preheat the oven to 350°F. In a greased baking dish, arrange the sliced apple and raspberries and pour the apple juice to cover this.
2. In a bowl, mix the rolled oats, sugar and spices to form a rough flour. To this, add the butter and mix in with your fingers to make the crumble topping.
3. Layer the crumble topping onto the laid out apples and raspberries until they are covered with a uniform layer.
4. Bake for about 45 – 60 minutes.
5. This crumble can be served hot or cold.

34.   Fudgy Sweet Potato Brownies

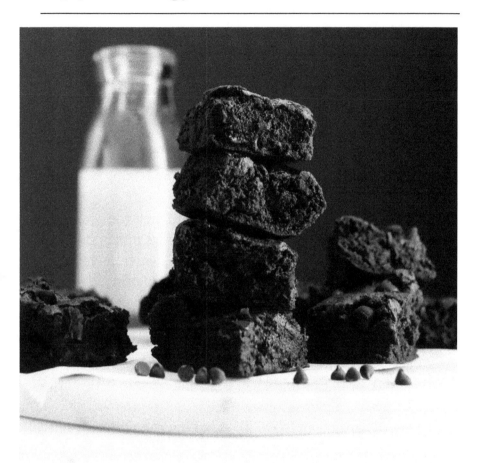

Prep Time:: 40 Minutes

Serves: 4

Ingredients:

- ¼ cup cold pressed Coconut Oil
- ¾ cup unsweetened Cocoa Powder

- ½ cup Pastry Flour (Whole Wheat preferred)
- 1 pinch Baking Powder
- 1 pinch fine Sea Salt
- 1 cup Coconut Sugar
- 1 cup Sweet Potato Puree
- 1 Tbsp. ground flaxseed meal + 3 Tbsp. cool water
- 1½ tsp pure vanilla extract

Directions:

1. In a small bowl, add the flour, salt and baking powder and mix well.
2. Place a saucepan on a low flame and melt the coconut oil. Stir in the cocoa powder until the entire mix is smooth.
3. Add the sweet potato, flax seed meal, water, sugar and vanilla to a large bowl and whisk thoroughly. You might need to keep at it for a bit as the coconut sugar can take a bit of time to dissolve.
4. Add the cocoa and coconut oil mixture to the large bowl and keep whisking.
5. Add flour to this and keep whisking till smooth and the batter has a glossy appearance.
6. Lightly grease an 8"x8" glass baking pan with coconut oil, and preheat the oven to 350°F.
7. Pour the batter into the pan, and bake for 20 to 30 minutes.
8. The top should appear hard and baked. When you stick a butter knife into the center, it should come out smooth with a few moist crumbs.
9. Note: The total baking time will depend on what type of sweet potatoes you use.
10. In case you use canned puree, it can take a bit longer as they have higher moisture content.

Stir in the flour till smooth, scrap into the prepared pan.

35. Millet Pancakes with Prune Compote

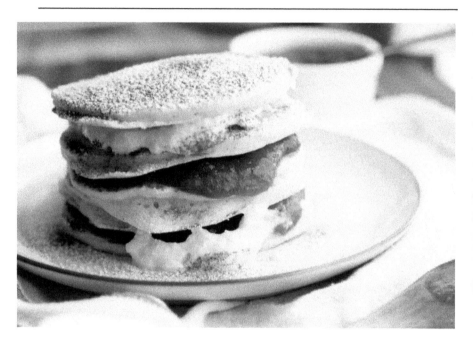

Yields 4: servings

Ingredients

- 2 tablespoons apple juice
- 2 tablespoons brown sugar
- 2 cups water
- 16 oz. organic dried plums pitted and softened.
- Vegetables cooking spray
- 2 tablespoons millet
- 1 egg, lightly beaten
- 1/3 cup plain non-fat yogurt
- 1 tablespoon sugar
- ½ cup carbonated water

- 1 teaspoon salt
- 2 cups skim milk
- 1 cup millet

Directions:

1. Place millet, milk, and salt in a medium saucepan and bring to boil, then simmer covered for 20 minutes.

2. Stir in the sugar, carbonated water, egg, yogurt, and millet flour.

3. Over medium heat, preheat a large non-stick skillet and spray with vegetable cooking spray.

4. Ladle batter into the skillet and spread with a spoon to form 3-inch pancakes. Fry until golden brown. Flip over and continue cooking for 4 minutes.

5. Place prunes, sugar, and water and apple juice in a saucepan and bring to a boil.

Reduce the heat and simmer for 12 minutes or until the prunes are tender.

6. Let the prune completely cool for a few minutes then serve on pancakes

36.   Nettle Crepes with Raspberries

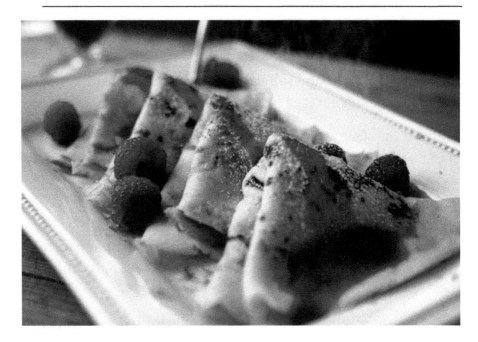

Yields: 2 servings

Ingredients

- Fresh raspberries
- Vegetable cooking spray
- 1 teaspoon salt
- ¼-teaspoon white pepper
- 7 oz. young nettle shots, blanched and chopped
- 1-cup all-purpose flour
- 2 cups organic milk
- 2 organic eggs

Directions:

1. In a medium bowl, beat the eggs; add nettle, milk, pepper, and salt. Whisk until well combined.

2. Preheat a large nonstick skillet over medium heat, and then spray with vegetable cooking spray.

3. Pour out 3 tablespoons of batter onto the skillet, rotating the skillet very quickly until

the bottom evenly coats. Cook the crepe for 2 minutes or until light brown. Flip and

cook for another 30 seconds then remove from the skillet.

4. Repeat step 3 until all the batter is finished.

5. Serve crepe with mashed raspberries.

Sauces, Condiments And Dressings

37. Cherry Coconut Porridge

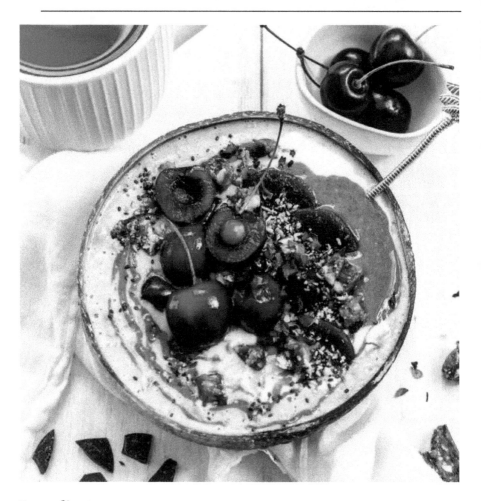

Ingredients

- 1.5cups oats
- 4 tablespoons chia seed
- 3-4cups of coconut drinking milk
- 3 tablespoons raw cacao
- pinch of stevia
- coconut shavings

- cherries (fresh or frozen)
- dark chocolate shavings
- maple syrup

Directions:

1. Combine oats, chia, coconut milk, cacao and stevia in a saucepan.

Bring to a boil over medium heat and then simmer over lower heat until oats are cooked.

2. Pour into a bowl and top with coconut shavings, cherries, dark chocolate shavings and maple syrup to taste.

38.   Maple, Walnut and Flaxseed Pancakes Recipe

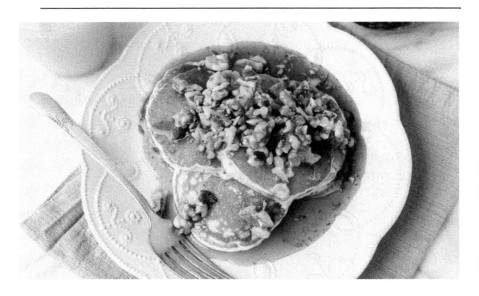

Ingredients:

- 1 cup all-purpose flour
- 1/4 cup flaxseed meal*
- 1/4 cup finely chopped walnuts
- 1 1/2 teaspoons baking powder
- 1/2 teaspoon baking soda
- 1/2 teaspoon salt
- 1 1/4 cups reduced-fat (2%) buttermilk
- 1/4 cup pure maple syrup
- 1 large egg
- 1 tablespoon (or more) vegetable oil
- Additional pure maple syrup

Directions:

1. Whisk flour, flaxseed meal, walnuts, baking powder, baking soda and salt in medium bowl. In a separate medium bowl, whisk buttermilk, 1/4 cup maple syrup and egg. Add buttermilk mixture to dry ingredients and whisk until incorporated.

2. Brush a large nonstick skillet lightly with vegetable oil and heat over medium heat. Working in batches, add batter to skillet by scant 1/4-cupfuls.

3. Cook, until bubbles appear on surface of pancakes and undersides, are golden brown, about 2 minutes.

4. Turn pancakes over and cook until golden on bottom, about 2 minutes. Brush skillet lightly with vegetable oil as needed between batches. Transfer pancakes to plates. Serve with additional maple syrup.

39.   Avocado Chocolate Mousse

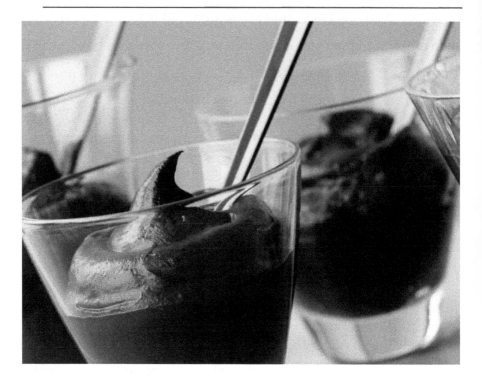

Ingredients

- 3 ripe avocados
- 6 oz plain Greek yoghurt
- 1 bar dark chocolate
- 1/8 cup unsweetened almond milk
- 1/4 cup finely ground espresso beans
- 2 tbsp raw honey
- 1 tsp vanilla extract
- 1/2 tsp sea salt
- 1/4 cup sugar

- 1/4 cup cocoa powder

Directions:

1. Mix all ingredients together, then puree in blender.

2. Set in fridge to cool.

40. Chocolate Cake with Vanilla Frosting

Ingredients:

For Cake:

- ½ teaspoon baking soda
- 12 free-range eggs
- 1 cup virgin coconut oil
- ½ cup raw cacao powder
- 1 cup coconut flour
- 1 cup pure maple syrup
- 4 tablespoons vanilla extract
- 1 teaspoon salt
- For Vanilla Icing:
- 2 cans of full-fat coconut cream (liquid drained from can)
- 4 tablespoons pure maple syrup
- ½ teaspoon almond extract
- 4 teaspoons vanilla extract

Directions:

For Cake:

1.Add all of the ingredients to a blender and blend on high for 30-45 seconds, allowing the eggs to froth.

2.Pour batter evenly into two 6 inch cake pans.

3.Bake at 350 degrees for 30 minutes or until cake passes the toothpick test.

4.Cool before frosting.

For Vanilla Icing:

1.Chill coconut milk in the fridge for at least 6 hours, preferably overnight. (Recipe will not work without it being chilled.)

2.Without shaking the cans, remove them from the refrigerator.

3.Carefully open the cans of coconut milk and scoop the thickened cream into a bowl.

4.Add the pure maple syrup, vanilla extract, and almond extract to the heavy coconut cream.

5.Mix thoroughly with a hand mixer... will take 3-5 minutes.

6.Place in refrigerator and allow icing to cool to thicken until it meets the texture you most prefer. Frost the cake.

Lightning Source UK Ltd.
Milton Keynes UK
UKHW020638140621
385477UK00005B/35